Rafael Bispo Paschoalini

Cytological criteria associated with the luminal phenotype of breast cancer

Rafael Bispo Paschoalini

Cytological criteria associated with the luminal phenotype of breast cancer

The luminal phenotype of breast cancer on fine needle aspiration biopsy (FNAB)

ScienciaScripts

Imprint

Cover image: www.ingimage.com

This book is a translation from the original published under ISBN 978-3-330-76343-2.

Publisher:
Sciencia Scripts
is a trademark of
Dodo Books Indian Ocean Ltd. and OmniScriptum S.R.L publishing group

120 High Road, East Finchley, London, N2 9ED, United Kingdom
Str. Armeneasca 28/1, office 1, Chisinau MD-2012, Republic of Moldova, Europe
Managing Directors: Ieva Konstantinova, Victoria Ursu
info@omniscriptum.com

Printed at: see last page
ISBN: 978-620-8-40543-4

Dedication

To my parents, Rodolfo and Valéria, and my brother, Lucas, for all the love and affection that motivated me to persevere towards this achievement.

To my grandparents Benito and Marylena, for their constant encouragement.

Thank you

To Prof Dr Rozany Mucha Dufloth for all her attention and patience, for her enthusiasm and encouragement.

To Prof Dr Fernando Carlos de Landèr Schmitt for his vote of confidence in carrying out this work.

To Dr Francisco Alves Moraes Neto for the opportunity to carry out this work in cooperation.

To Dr Cleverson Teixeira Soares for his valuable learning and constant encouragement.

To all the friends, teachers and staff of the Department of Pathology and the Postgraduate Programme at UNESP.

"And you took off your glasses and put them on Miguilim, with all your might.

Look now!

Miguilim looked. He couldn't believe it! Everything was bright, everything new and beautiful and different, the things, the trees, the people's faces.

I saw little grains of sand, the skin of the earth, the smallest pebbles, the little ants walking on the ground from a distance.

And I was dizzy. Here, there, my God, so much (...).

My heart was pounding."

João Guimarães Rosa - *in* Campo Geral, Manuelzão e Miguilim.

Summary

INTRODUCTION: Breast carcinoma is a heterogeneous disease. It can be categorised into phenotypes, with different prognoses, based on the expression of certain proteins. The luminal phenotype is the most common, accounting for around 70% of cases, and specific treatments for this phenotype of breast carcinoma are already being studied, with a promising improvement in the prognosis of affected patients. However, cytological criteria that could predict this phenotype in material obtained by fine needle aspiration biopsy (FNAB) have yet to be defined. OBJECTIVE: To investigate individual cytological criteria present in FNAB that may be associated with the diagnosis of the luminal phenotype of breast carcinoma. METHODS: This is a cross-sectional study with a descriptive and comparative component. FNAC slides and specimens of invasive ductal and lobular breast carcinomas from 2000 to 2009 were selected from the archive of the Pathology Laboratory of the Amaral Carvalho Hospital in Jaú/São Paulo, totalling 297 cases. Cylinders 2mm in diameter were extracted from the donor blocks and deposited in the recipient paraffin blocks using *Tissue Microarrays* (Bencher Instruments®, Silver Spring, Maryland). These sections were immunohistochemically analysed to differentiate breast carcinoma phenotypes according to the Molecular Classification. The slides obtained by FNAC were reviewed under a multi-observation microscope (BX50 Olympus®, Japan) by two pathologists (RMD and FMN), and the five cytological criteria were studied individually: cellularity, cell cohesion, necrosis, nucleoli and nuclear atypia. Fisher's exact test was used to test the association between cytological criteria and breast carcinoma phenotypes.

RESULTS: Of the 297 cases selected, 169 were included, resulting in the following phenotypes - luminal A: 107 (63.3%), luminal B: 39 (23.1%), HER2 overexpression: 8 (4.7%), and triple negative: 15 (8.9%). The cytological criteria that were associated with the luminal phenotype were: low or moderate cellularity (40.4%) (OR = 7.12, 95%CI: 1.61 - 31.52), inconspicuous or non-prominent nucleoli (55.5%) (OR = 8.31, 95%CI: 2.36 - 29.19) and mild or moderate nuclear atypia (44.5%) (OR = 8.42, 95%CI: 1.90 - 37.25). The cytological criteria associated with luminal phenotype A were: inconspicuous or present non-prominent nucleoli (62.6%) (OR = 2.99, 95%CI: 1.39 - 6.41), minor loss of cell cohesion (OR = 0.46, 95%CI: 0.24 - 0.88), showing clusters with moderate to intense cell cohesion, and absence of necrosis (40.2%) (OR = 0.32, 95%CI: 0.15 - 0.68). CONCLUSION: The cytological criteria present in the slides obtained by FNAB and most associated with the luminal phenotype of breast carcinoma were low and moderate cellularity, inconspicuous or non-prominent nucleoli and mild to moderate nuclear atypia. It is worth noting that for luminal phenotype A, the cytological criteria that were most associated were: inconspicuous or present non-prominent nucleoli, moderate to intense cell cohesion and absence of necrosis. Distinguishing the luminal phenotype is of clinical relevance, as it has a better prognosis, related to lower mortality and lower metastasis rates.

Summary

CHAPTER 1

Introduction

Breast carcinoma is the most common malignant neoplasm in women of all ethnic groups, with the exception of non-melanoma skin tumours, accounting for around 25% of all cancer cases worldwide (approximately 1.4 million new cases). In 2017, 252,710 new cases of the neoplasm were estimated in women in the United States (ACS, 2017). In Brazil, data for 2016 indicated more than 57,960 new cases, with an incidence rate of 56.20 cases per 100,000 women, and it is still the most incident neoplasm in women in all regions (except in the North, where cervical cancer remains the most frequent), and the leading cause of cancer death in women in the country (15.7 per cent of all deaths), ranking fifth in overall cancer mortality, with 458,000 deaths (INCA, 2015).

Breast carcinoma mortality rates decreased between 2007 and 2011, with a drop of 3.2 per cent per year in white women and 2.4 per cent per year in black women under the age of 50; in women aged 50 and over, the decrease was 1.8 per cent per year in white women and 1.1 per cent per year in black women (Kohler et al, 2015). The reduction in mortality is mainly attributable to improvements in early detection, effective treatment and a reduction in incidence, associated with the decline in the use of hormone replacement therapies during the menopause. Even so, there were an estimated 40,610 deaths from breast carcinoma in women in the United States in 2017 (ACS, 2017). In Brazil, this figure was 14,206 deaths (INCA, 2015).

In order to reduce mortality from this neoplasm, which is still high, researchers are keen to better characterise breast carcinoma in order to predict its biological behaviour, ensure more appropriate treatment and improve patients' prognosis.

In view of the great heterogeneity of breast carcinoma cases, especially in relation to the varied clinical outcomes, there has been extensive study of the gene expression profile (Naderi et al. 2007; Sotiriou et aL, 2006; Sorlie et al., 2003; Van't Veer et al., 2002; Sorlie et al. 2001; Perou et aL, 2000) in order to identify a molecular signature for each type of tumour. In this context, it is worth highlighting the work of the Stanford group, which demonstrated that the phenotypic diversity of breast carcinomas was accompanied by a corresponding diversity in gene expression (Sorlie et aL, 2003; Sorlie et aL, 2001; Perou et al., 2000).

The classification of breast carcinomas into molecular phenotypes can predict how they respond to specific therapeutic agents, and it is important to differentiate them as early as possible. Within this context, fine-needle aspiration biopsy (FNAB), combined with clinical and imaging tests, is a widely accepted diagnostic method, both in clinical studies and in routine diagnosis, enabling early diagnosis of breast carcinoma in around 80% of cases (Kocjan et aL, 2008; Koss, 2003; Koss, 1993).

It is well known that for the initial investigation of breast lesions suspected of being malignant, by physical examination or imaging tests, there are various diagnostic modalities that can be used. Strictly speaking, the selection of the biopsy approach method will depend on the clinical circumstances, the imaging findings, the skill of the test operator and the doctor's confidence in carrying it out (Karimzadeh et al., 2008). The main diagnostic methods used are: fine needle aspiration biopsy (FNAB), percutaneous biopsy and open surgical biopsy (excisional or incisional) (Chaiwun et al., 2007; Stanley et al., 2000).

Since its introduction by Martin and Ellis in 1930 (Martin et al., 1930), FNAB has been used to obtain samples for cytological diagnosis in various organs, and is a routine procedure for assessing breast lesions. In most institutions, FNAB has been the initial method for investigating abnormalities diagnosed by mammography (Kocjan et al., 2006).

Among the advantages of FNAB, we can mention that it is a fast, low-cost diagnostic method - as it does not require anaesthesia or hospitalisation - and involves less morbidity, due to lower post-procedure risks (Zagorianakou et aL, 2005; Layfield et aL, 1993). When guided by ultrasound, studies show a sensitivity of around 90 per cent and specificity of around 100 per cent compared to non-image-guided FNAB (Kamphausen et aL, 2003; Arisio et aL, 1998). It is also worth noting, according to some studies, that when the slide is read by an experienced cytopathologist, better diagnostic accuracy is obtained, with sensitivity ranging from 60 to 93% and specificity of around 100% (Karimzadeh et al., 2008; Arisio et al., 1998; Eisenberg et al., 1986).

As for the cytological criteria for diagnosing breast carcinoma in FNAB smears, at least three must be present: marked cellularity, cell dissociation and atypia. Most carcinomas present an abundant population of neoplastic cells, predominantly dispersed and isolated. They can also present in three-dimensional cell aggregates with greater cell cohesion, in fewer cases with a lower degree of cell dissociation. Cytological atypia, in turn, consists of one or more of the following criteria: high nucleus/cytoplasm ratio, increased nucleus size, pleomorphism, anisokaryosis, coarsely granular chromatin, hyperchromasia, conspicuous, irregular or multiple nucleoli (Bibbo, et al. 2008; DeMay, 2007; Koss et aL, 2006).

Cytologically, invasive ductal carcinoma is characterised by smears with marked cellularity, either with cells arranged in isolation or in three-dimensional aggregates, syncytial groupings and occasional glandular-s/7n//e arrangements, with obvious atypia when of high nuclear grade, which does not occur in those of low nuclear grade. Therefore, the diagnosis of high nuclear grade breast carcinomas in FNAB smears has better accuracy and agreement among cytopathologists (Lakhani et al., 2012; Bibbo et al., 2008).

On the other hand, invasive lobular carcinoma, particularly the classic type, has been reported to be difficult to diagnose, showing smears with low cellularity, small cells with small, relatively uniform nuclei, groups of cells without obvious pleomorphism and which can be interpreted as a benign lesion (Dufloth et al, 2015; Lakhani et al, 2012; Koss et al, 2006; Hwang et al, 2004; Tan et al, 2002). In addition, it is known that there is a tendency for cells to form small rows - the "Indian rows" - with characteristically very small nuclei, and this cytological criterion is a very useful clue for this diagnosis (Kocjan et al., 2008; DeMay, 2007). However, this cytological criterion is not always present. Other cytological criteria mentioned for the nucleus are the irregularity of the nuclear membrane and the presence of cracks or furrows. Occasionally, a target-like intracytoplasmic lumen and cells with a signet ring appearance can be seen (Lakhani et aL, 2012).

In this context, it is clear that cytological smears obtained by FNAB are less accurate in the cytological diagnosis of lobular carcinoma than in the case of ductal carcinoma (Shabb et aL, 2013).

It is important to point out that therapeutic planning is carried out preoperatively and takes into account the results obtained from FNAB. It is important to gather as much information as possible from cytological specimens, since histological type, tumour grade, hormone receptor *status* and cell proliferation rate, which are prognostic indicators, can be assessed using this method. With regard to hormone *status*, studies show that diagnostic agreement ranges from 80% to 90% between the surgical specimen and the sample obtained by FNAB. The proliferation index estimated by Ki67 has significant prognostic value and is independent of factors such as the presence of axillary invasion, hormonal *status* and tumour size, and can also be assessed in cytological samples (Marinsec et aL 2013; Jayaram et aL, 2005; Lõfgren et aL, 2003; Billgren et aL, 2002).

Currently, genomic studies based on cDNA *microarray* techniques carried out on material obtained by FNAC allow everything from the identification of patients at high risk of developing breast carcinoma to tumour characterisation and prediction of the disease's response to treatment, in order to assess sensitivity to chemotherapy (Schmittet aL, 2012; DiLorito et aL, 2011; Tabchy et aL, 2010; Schmitt et aL, 2007).

In line with the advances in knowledge of the molecular biology of breast carcinoma, a notable contribution to translational research was the characterisation of different gene expression profiles in breast carcinoma in a study carried out by Perou and his team, which used a platform of 8,100 genes in around 65 samples belonging to 42 patients (Perou et aL, 2000).

The first level of classification separated carcinomas negative for oestrogen receptors (RE-) and carcinomas positive for the expression of this receptor (RE+). Subsequently, *breast* carcinomas were classified into five distinct molecular phenotypes: luminal A (RE+ and *Human epithelial receptor 2* [HER2]-), luminal B (RE+ and HER2+), basal (RE HER2- and cytokeratins [CKs] 5/6+ and CK17+), HER2 overexpression (RE- and HER2+) and *normal breast-like* (Sorlie et aL, 2001).

The extensive knowledge gained from studies of gene expression profiles in breast carcinoma over the last 15 years has enabled the configuration of the classification of molecular phenotypes based on semi-quantitative scores of immunohistochemical markers, including the cell proliferation index expressed by Ki67 and the expression of the progesterone receptor (PR) as auxiliary classification criteria (Aleksandarany et aL 2012; Goldhirsch et aL, 2011; Callagy et aL 2003;).

The classification of breast carcinoma based on the 12[i/?] St *Gallen International Breast Cancer Conference* in 2011 was highlighted for defining the classification of the following breast carcinoma phenotypes: luminal A (RE+ and/or RP+, low Ki67 and HER2-), luminal B (RE+ and/or RP+, high Ki67 and/or HER2+), HER2 overexpression (RE-, RP- and HER2+) and triple negative (RE-, RP-, HER2-) (Goldhirsch et aL, 2011).

In the following conferences, with the growing interest in better characterising the A and B luminal phenotypes, both the cell proliferation index and progesterone receptor positivity thresholds were revised. Until then, the value used as a *cut-off* for Ki67, based on review studies, was 14% for defining tumours with a low or high proliferation index. Currently, Ki67 of 20% has been accepted as the threshold between low and high cell proliferation (Petrelli et al. 2015; Sato et al., 2014). The clinicopathological terms 'luminal *A-*

like' and 'luminal *B-like'* were also categorised, corresponding to the luminal A and luminal B molecular phenotypes, respectively (Maisonneuve et al., 2014).

The 2015 consensus of the *14th St Gallen International Breast Cancer Conference* considers that among hormone receptor-positive breast carcinomas, the luminal A and luminal B phenotypes account for approximately 60% to 70% of breast carcinomas (Coates et al., 2015; Esposito et al., 2015).

Through the *St Gallen* classification and supported by a publication from the *Cancer Genome Atlas Network*, luminal phenotype carcinomas were highlighted as being the most heterogeneous in terms of gene expression, mutation spectrum and gene copy number alterations, and therefore with a variable clinical prognosis (CGAN, 2012).

The luminal A phenotype was characterised by the high expression of genes represented by luminal epithelial cells, for example the cytokeratins (CK) CK7, CK8, CK18 and CK19. This phenotype is associated with a lower histological grade, a lower proliferation rate cell and a genetic signature with a better prognosis, with a generally satisfactory response to antiestrogen therapy, since it has high endocrine sensitivity (CGAN, 2012; Blows et al., 2010).

The luminal B phenotype was characterised by low or moderate expression of genes expressed by luminal epithelial cells, such as CK7, CK8, CK18 and CK19, as well as lower expression of progesterone receptors, a high rate of cell proliferation and a higher histological grade. This phenotype is associated with a worse prognosis, and is particularly related to tumour recurrence as it has possible similarities with RE - tumours (HER2 overexpression and triple negative phenotypes), and chemotherapy is recommended in addition to endocrine therapy (CGAN, 2012; Cheang et aL, 2009).

The distinction between luminal phenotypes in the clinical context is becoming more relevant. In terms of clinical risk, their association with high body mass index and reproductive factors has been identified in patients with ER+ breast carcinoma (Xiaohong R et aL, 2010). The study of imaging methods may also prove useful in distinguishing the luminal phenotype (Zhang et aL, 2015; Pessoa, 2014). These advances are directly related to the growing understanding of the diverse biological behaviour associated with prognostic and predictive factors of luminal carcinomas (Aleksandarany et aL 2012; CGAN, 2012; Lowery et aL 2012).

The distinction between luminal A and luminal B phenotypes is also relevant. Luminal B breast carcinomas do not show corresponding expression of oestrogen-regulated genes, so they may be associated with alternative growth pathways (Geyer et aL 2012; Creighton, 2012). At a molecular level, they are extremely different from luminal phenotype A carcinomas in terms of gene expression, gene copy number, somatic mutations and DNA methylation (CGAN, 2012). It is known that luminal phenotype B carcinomas have a wider range of genetic and genomic alterations than those of luminal phenotype A, which has been the subject of extensive research (Bartsch et aL,2013).

With regard to the study of target therapies, there are several chemotherapies for the luminal phenotype. Particularly in relation to the B phenotype, alterations to the *phosphoinositide 3-kinase / mammalian target of rapamycin* (PI3K/mTOR), *fibroblast growth factor receptor* (FGFR) and *cyclin dependent kinase 4/6* (CDK4/6) inhibition pathways have been described (Bartsch et aL, 2013). Some of these agents are in phase I and II studies, such as TKI235 - Dovitinib, an FGFR inhibitor - in cases of progression of breast carcinomas with RE + receptors. Everolimus is an oral mTOR inhibitor that has already been approved, in combination with Exemestane, for the treatment of cases of metastatic breast carcinoma, RE+ and refractory to other therapies (Esposito et al, 2015; Creighton, 2012; Baselga et aL 2012).

An association between the luminal phenotype and the lobular histological subtype of breast carcinoma has been described (Ciriello et al, 2015). In a series of 817 cases containing 127 invasive lobular carcinomas, it was shown that these tumours, in addition to loss of E-cadherin expression, also had mutations involving *phosphatase and tensin homolog* (PTEN), *T-box transcription factor 3* (TBX3) and *forkhead box protein A1* (FOXA1), and were mainly associated with the luminal A phenotype. PTEN inactivation was shown to be a discriminating feature of these carcinomas compared to invasive ductal carcinoma with luminal A phenotype. Also, the lower expression of oestrogen receptors in lobular carcinoma with luminal phenotype A could determine a better response to aromatase inhibitors such as Letrozole, compared to Tamoxifen (Ciriello et aL, 2015; Sikora, 2014).

In relation to systemic treatment decisions for patients with breast carcinoma, a recent Swedish study correlated the molecular phenotype of the primary tumour with that of synchronous metastases in the axillary lymph nodes of 85 patients, finding greater chances of distant metastasis and death in all molecular phenotypes, compared to luminal A (Falk et aL, 2013). These data reinforce the relevance of identifying the luminal phenotype in order to seek better therapeutic planning.

In relation to the variable prognosis of breast carcinoma, the triple negative phenotype is characterised by greater aggressiveness, lower survival rates and a relationship with hereditary breast carcinoma, mostly comprising the basal-Z/ke molecular subtype (Bose, 2015; Rakha et aL, 2008; Banerjee et aL, 2006). It is also possible to characterise the basal phenotype in the clinical context by immunoreactivity for basal or myoepithelial cell markers, generally applying a combination of high molecular weight cytokeratins (CK5/6, CK14, CK17) and EGFR. The association of this phenotype with mutations in the BRCA1 gene and the p53 tumour suppressor gene makes it possible to use poly(ADP-ribose) polymerase inhibitors (PARP inhibitors) (Bose, 2015; Badve et aL, 2011; Fadare et aL, 2007).

In view of the advances made in understanding the molecular biology of breast carcinoma, the cytological characterisation of molecular phenotypes in FNAB material is relevant. Cytologically, the characterisation of the basal phenotype was explored and the cytological criterion 'necrosis' was found to be present in 67.4% of the smears obtained by FNAB in basal phenotype breast carcinomas. It is also worth highlighting the presence of the cytological criteria 'greater cellularity' and 'prominent nucleoli' in this phenotype compared to the luminal A phenotype, demonstrating that these were the cytological criteria most associated with the basal phenotype of breast carcinoma (Dufloth et aL, 2009).

The luminal phenotype, however, despite being the most common, with the best prognosis and promising advances in target therapies, still lacks the cytological characterisation described. Using FNAC samples and immunohistochemical results obtained by the *tissue microarray* (TMA) technique from invasive ductal and lobular breast carcinomas, the aim of this study was to investigate the cytological criteria individually present in FNAC smears that could indicate the luminal phenotype of breast carcinoma.

CHAPTER 2

Objectives

2.1. General objective

To investigate the individual cytological criteria present in cytological smears obtained by fine needle aspiration and which could indicate the luminal phenotype of breast carcinoma, using a series of breast carcinomas classified according to the current molecular classification as the gold standard, by means of an immunohistochemical study using the *tissue microarray* (TMA) technique.

2.2. Specific objectives

1. To verify the frequency of the individual cytological criteria present in the cytological smears obtained by FNAB in relation to the molecular phenotypes of breast carcinoma.
2. To analyse the association between the individual cytological criteria present in the cytological smears obtained by FNAB and the diagnosis of the luminal phenotype of breast carcinoma.

CHAPTER 3

Methods

3.1. Type of study

This was a cross-sectional study, with a descriptive and comparative component, as part of the research line in Oncopathology of the Postgraduate Programme in Pathology at the Universidade Estadual Paulista "Júlio de Mesquita Filho" (UNESP), Botucatu/São Paulo - Brazil, in collaboration with the Faculty of Medicine of the University of Porto/Portugal. The study was a sub-project of the project entitled "Analysis of the clinical relevance of the histological classification of lobular and ductal breast carcinomas and its relationship with the molecular classification of the luminal type", CEP protocol No. 10/2012.

3.2. Selection of subjects

3.2.1. Inclusion criteria

The study included 297 cases of patients over the age of 18 with a diagnosis of breast carcinoma - lobular or ductal - confirmed by histological study of the biopsy or operative specimen, with FNAB having been performed prior to the biopsy or excision of the tumour. The cases were selected at the Pathology Laboratory of the Amaral Carvalho Hospital in Jaú.

3.2.2. Exclusion criteria

We excluded 128 cases whose slides and/or blocks could not be found or did not have the technical conditions to assess protein expression using immunohistochemistry.

3.3. Variables under study

Figura A independent

The independent variables were five pre-established individual cytological criteria: cellularity, cell cohesion, necrosis, nucleolus and nuclear atypia. These five cytological criteria are summarised in Table 1 and shown in the figures (Figures A-F) and were analysed individually through microscopic review of cytological smears obtained by FNAB, using an optical microscope for multiple observers (BX50 Olympus®, Japan). The independent variables were analysed in a blinded (double-blind) manner in relation to the breast carcinoma phenotype obtained in each case (dependent variable) (see below).

Figura B dependent riables

Breast carcinoma phenotypes were the dependent variables and followed the Perou classification (Perou et aL, 2000), modified by Sorlie (Sorlie et aL, 2001) and reviewed at the *13th St Gallen International Breast Cancer Conference* (Maisonneuve et aL, 2014; Goldhirsch et aL 2011), which include characterisation of the luminal phenotype (Table 2).

Table 1 - Independent variables

Variable	Definition	Categorisation
Cellularity	Number of cells in the smear	1- **- Discreet** 2- **Moderate** 3- **Accentuated**
Cell cohesion	Degree of cell association	1- Predominance of aggregated cells: **marked** cell cohesion 2- Equal representation of aggregated cells and dissociated cells: **moderate** cell cohesion 3- Predominance of dissociated cells: **little** cell **cohesion**
Necrosis	Presence of areas of necrosis	1 - **Presence** of necrosis 2- **Absence of** necrosis
Nucleolus	Appearance of the nucleolus	1- **Inconspicuous nucle**olus or micronucleolus only: inconspicuous nucleolus 2- Isolated macronucleus **present** in most cells: nucleolus present 3- Multiple macronucleoli present: nucleolus **present and prominent**

Nuclear atypia	Nuclear pleomorphism	1- - **Absent** 2- **Discreet** 3- **Moderate** 4- **Intense**

SOURCES: DeMay M. Practical principies of cytopathology. Revised Edition. American Society for Clinical Pathology. 2007; Koss LG. Diagnostic Cytology and its histopathologic bases, 5th ed., vol. 1, 2006.

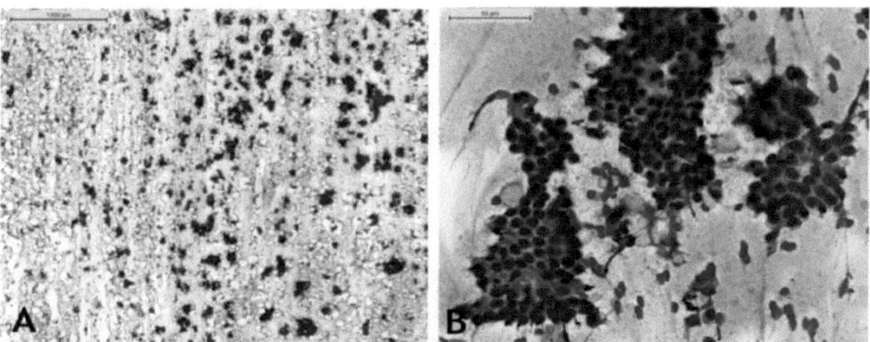

Figura C - Marked cellularity (May-Grunwald Giemsa, x50).
Figura D - Strong cohesion (HE, x400).

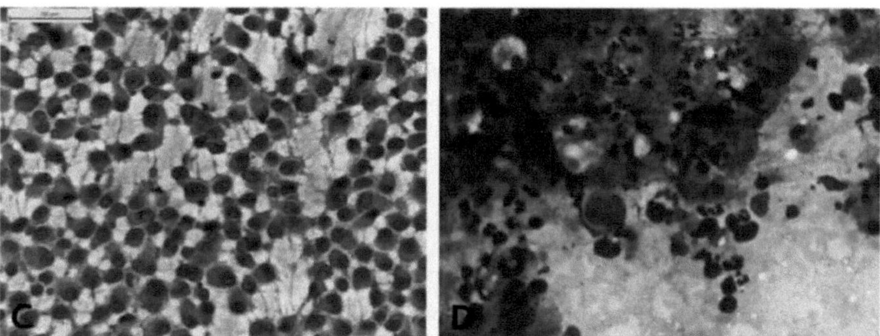

Figura E - Poorly cohesive cells (HE, x400).
Figura F - Presence of necrosis (May-Grunwald Giemsa, x400).

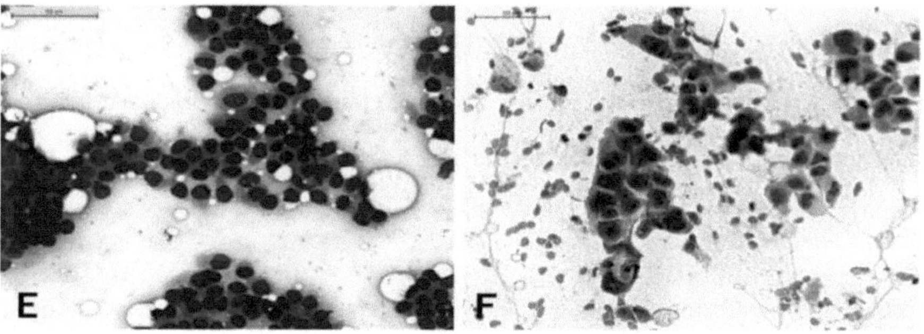

Figura G - No necrosis (May-Grunwald Giemsa, x400).
Figura H - Prominent nucleoli and intense cytological atypia (Pap, x400).

Table 2 - Dependent variables: Molecular classification of breast carcinoma.

Molecular phenotype	RE	PR	HER2	Ki67
Luminal A	+	+	-	< 20%
Luminal B	+	+/-	-	> 20%
	+	+/-	+	Any
HER2 overexpression	-	-	+	Any
Triple-negative	-	-	-	Any

ER (Oestrogen Receptor); PR (Progesterone *Receptor*); HER2 *(Human Epidermal Growth Factor Receptor 2);* Ki67 (Cell Proliferation Index) SOURCE: St *Gallen Consensus Conference* 2013.

3.4. Data collection

All the copies of the cytopathological and anatomopathological reports issued by the pathologists at the Pathology Laboratory of the Amaral Carvalho Hospital, Jaú/São Paulo, between 2000 and 2009 were identified and separated. The slides and the respective paraffin blocks were stored in the laboratory and were removed from the archive for the analyses in this study. To build the sample, all the cases available in the laboratory were identified sequentially.

3.5. Data processing

3.5.1. Cytological criteria

The slides of the cytological smears of the material obtained by FNAB were previously fixed and stained using the HE, Papanicolaou and May-Grunwald Giemsa methods - following the protocols of the Pathology Laboratory of the Amaral Carvalho Hospital at Jaú /SP (Chart 3) (Marsan et al. 2001), and were reassessed by two pathologists (R.M.D. and F.A.N.M.) to identify the presence of five pre-established individual cytological criteria: cellularity, cell cohesion, necrosis, nucleolus and nuclear atypia (DeMay, 2007; Koss, 2006) (Table 1 and Figures A-F).

Chart 3 - Methods for fixing the material obtained by FNAB.

Colouring	Fastening method
HE	Immediately, in 95° alcohol
Pap smear	Immediately, in 95° alcohol
May-Grunwald-Giemsa	Air drying

SOURCE: Marsan C. Cytopathologie mammaire par ponction. Le pathologiste. Elsevier. 2001.

3.5.2. *Tissue Microarray* Technique (TMA)

The expression of all the immunohistochemical markers was studied using the TMA technique, following the protocols of the Institute of Molecular Pathology and Immunology of the University of Porto (IPATIMUP) (Gerhard et al., 2013).

Slides were obtained from the donor tissue blocks, from which two morphologically significant areas of carcinoma were selected. These slides were superimposed on the donor blocks and the two areas were marked on each one to delimit the material extraction site. Two 2 mm diameter cylinders were extracted from each donor block and placed in the previously prepared recipient blocks. The TMA receptor blocks were built on the *Tissue Microarray builder ab1802* (Abcam®, Cambridge, UK), consisting of a 24-cylinder mould and a *punch-extractor* syringe. Once all the cylinders had been deposited, the receiving blocks were the TMAs. Cases were placed in each receiving block to serve as internal controls (1 fragment of testicular tissue and 3 fragments of normal breast tissue). These samples were processed in the same way, as they belonged to the TMA. After sequential cutting to a thickness of 2 pm, the slides were wrapped in a layer of paraffin until they were used in the immunohistochemistry (IHQ) process. The first section of each TMA was stained with Haematoxylin-Eosin (HE) for morphological control of the presence of carcinoma. A cold plate (Leica® 11 EG1130, Germany) and a microtome (Reichet-Jung® 2030, Bicut, Germany) were used to make the histological sections. Two types of slides were used, depending on whether the histological sections were destined for HE staining (Marienfeld, Germany) or immunohistochemistry (Superfrost®Plus, Germany), the latter having greater adhesion power.

3.5.3. Immunohistochemistry (IHC) technique

Research into the expression of the immunohistochemical markers studied was carried out at the Immunohistochemistry Laboratory of the Pathology Department of the Amaral Carvalho Hospital in Jaú/SP (Neto FAM, 2014) using a manual immunohistochemical technique on the slides obtained by the TMA technique (except for the E-cadherin marker, conventional histological sections were used), following the institution's protocol and described briefly below: adhesive-coated slides suitable for immunohistochemical staining (SuperfrostOPlus, Germany) containing 3p histological sections from each TMA block were made, deparaffinised in an oven at 58°C for three hours, rehydrated in three 5' baths in xylene, two baths in 96% alcohol and two more baths in 70% alcohol and submitted to the antigen recovery technique using a Pascal® Dako pressure cooker (USA) in citrate buffer solution pH 7 (Target® Dako) or EDTA pH 8 for 45'. The slides were then incubated with the primary monoclonal antibodies for 30'. The clones, manufacturers, dilutions and recovery methods used are described in Table 4.

Chart 4 - Antibodies used in the immunohistochemical study.

Antibody	Clone	Dilution	Manufacturer	Recovery
E-cadherin	NCH-38	1:100	Dako	Citrate pH6
RE	SP1	1:100	Spring	Citrate pH6
PR	SP42	1:200	Spring	Citrate pH6
HER2	SP3	1:200	Spring	Citrate pH6
Ki67	MIB-1	1:200	Dako	EDTA

SOURCE: Neto FAM, 2014 Analysis of the clinical relevance of the histological classification of lobular breast carcinomas and its relationship with the molecular classification [master's thesis] UNESP - Hospital Amaral Carvalho de Jaú / SP protocol.

After incubation with the primary antibodies, the slides were washed in buffered saline solution (PBS) and incubated with Histofine® Universal Immuno-peroxidase Polymer, Anti-Mouse and - Rabbit (Nichirei, Tokyo, Japan) for 30'. The slides were washed again in PBS and incubated with Diaminobenzidine (DAB, Dako, USA) for 1' to reveal the immunohistochemical reaction and counterstained with haematoxylin (30"). External positive and negative controls (omission of the primary antibody) were included to validate the immunohistochemical reaction.

For the E-cadherin marker, membrane marking of any intensity on tumour cells was considered positive.

For the ER and PR markers, nuclear staining of any intensity in > 1% of tumour cells was considered positive, as recommended by ASCO/CAP *(American Society of Clinical Oncology/College of American Pathologists)* (Hammond et al., 2010). For *HER2*, the criteria established by ASCO-CAP (Wolff et al. 2013) and described in Table 5 were also used.

Chart 5 - Criteria established by ASCO-CAP for HER2.

HER2	Description
Score 0	No staining observed or incomplete and weak/weak membrane staining in < 10% of invasive tumour cells
Score 1 +	Incomplete and weak/poorly perceptible membrane staining in > 10% of invasive tumour cells.
Score 2+	Incomplete circumferential membrane staining and/or weak/moderate in > 10% of invasive tumour cells; or complete and intense circumferential membrane staining in < 10% of invasive tumour cells.
Score 3+	Complete and intense circumferential membrane staining in > 10% of invasive tumour cells

SOURCE: ASCO-CAP Test Guideline 2013 (Wolff et al. 2013).

The Ki67 cell proliferation index was determined by counting with a graduated reticle inserted into the eyepiece of an optical microscope (BX50 Olympus®, Japan), considering the percentage of cells showing nuclear staining of any intensity in 100 tumour cells in the most proliferative area ("hot spot"). The 20% *cut-off*, recently recommended by the *13th St Gallen Consensus Conference* 2013, was used to divide cases with a low cell proliferation index (< 20%) and a high cell proliferation index (>20%) (Maisonneuve et aL, 2014).

The tumours were classified according to the molecular classification *(St Gallen Consensus Conference* 2013) (Maisonneuve et aL, 2014) into the four phenotypes shown in Table 2 (above).

All slides were examined independently by two *senior* pathologists (R.D. and F.A.M.N.). Differences in interpretation were resolved using an optical microscope for multiple observers (BX50 Olympus®, Japan).

3.5.3. Fluorescence *in situ* hybridisation (FISH)

HER2 cases with a score of 2+ were submitted to the FISH test for HER2 gene amplification, as recommended by ASCO-CAP (Wolff et aL 2013), following the protocol of the Institute of Molecular Pathology and Immunology of the University of Porto (IPATIMUP) (Schmitt et aL, 1997). The HER2 FISH® *kit* (Dako, USA) was used. The histological sections were deparaffinised and rehydrated as described above for immunohistochemistry. The slides were then immersed for 3' in the *kit*'s wash buffer solution and incubated in a 95° water bath with the pre-treatment solution from the same *kit* for 10'. The slides were then washed in the buffer solution (two 3' baths at room temperature). The excess buffer solution was removed and 5 to 8 drops of Pepsin were applied to the histological sections and incubated for 10' at room temperature. The slides were washed again with the buffer solution (2 baths of 3' at room temperature), dehydrated in three solutions of 70%, 85% and 96% alcohol for 2' each and left to dry in the open air. 10 pL of the DNA probe was applied and the coverslip and sealant were placed around the periphery of the coverslip. The slides were then placed in the hybridiser (Hibridizer® Dako, USA) and subjected to a denaturation programme at 82° for 5' and overnight hybridisation (18 hours) at 45°. Removal of the sealant and coverslip and incubation with the *kit*'s stringency solution at 65° for 10'. The slides were washed in the buffer solution (2 baths of 3' at room temperature), dehydrated in three graduated solutions of 70%, 85% and 96% alcohol for 2' each, dried in the open air and finally 15pL of the fluorescent DAPI mounting medium that comes with the *kit* was applied and the slide covered with a coverslip for reading under a fluorescence microscope.

Two red and green DNA probes were used, corresponding to HER2 and the centromere of chromosome 17 (CEN-17) respectively. It was considered amplified when the HER2/CEN-17 ratio was equal to two or, if less than two, when there was a number of HER2 copies greater than or equal to six per cell, as recommended by ASCO-CAP (Wolff et al. 2013).

3.6. Statistical analysis

The statistical analysis of the magnitude of the association between the individual cytological criteria of the cytological smears obtained by FNAB and the diagnoses of breast carcinoma phenotypes, obtained using the TMA technique, was carried out using estimated *odds ratio* values with the respective 95% confidence intervals (95%CI). The data was described in absolute frequencies (n) and relative frequencies (%) to assess the association of cytological criteria. The *odds ratio* (OR) was considered significant when it did not include the value of 1. The analysis of the association of cytological criteria in predicting the diagnosis of the luminal phenotype of breast carcinoma was carried out using logistic regression models, including all the criteria, using *backward* selection. The results of the logistic regression analysis were expressed as OR values, with the respective 95%CI. These criteria were compared between breast carcinoma phenotypes using Fisher's exact test. The significance level assumed was 5% and the software used for the statistical analysis was SAS, Version 9.2.

3.7. Ethical aspects

The precepts of the Code of Medical Ethics were followed for the use of patient data and the principles set out in Resolutions no. 196/96, no. 251/97 of the National Health Council and the rules of the UNESP Research Ethics Committee (Protocol 4117-2012; Of.23/2014-CEP) were respected.

CHAPTER 4

Results

Of the total of 297 cases selected for this study, 169 cases were included. After complete immunohistochemical evaluation of the TMA slides, applying the molecular classification of phenotypes accepted by the *13?ʰ St Gallen Consensus Conference,* the following phenotypes were identified: 107 luminal A (63.3%), 39 luminal B (23.1%), 8 HER2 overexpression (4.7%) and 15 triple negative (8.9%) (Table 2). 146 cases were RE+ (86.4%) and therefore classified as luminal phenotype (Table 3).

Frequency analysis and association of individual criteria present in FNAB samples showed that diagnosis of the luminal phenotype of breast carcinoma was indicated by mild/moderate cellularity (40.4%) (OR = 7.12, 95% CI: 1.61 - 31.52), inconspicuous or present non-prominent nucleoli (55.5%) (OR = 8.31, 95% CI: 2.36 - 29.19) and mild/moderate nuclear atypia (44.5%) (OR = 8.42, 95% CI: 1.90-37.25).

Inconspicuous or present non-prominent nucleoli (62.6%) (OR = 4.43, 95% CI: 2.24 - 8.77), moderate or intense cell cohesion (54.2%) (OR = 0.46, 95% CI: 0.24 - 0.88), and absence of necrosis (40.2%) (OR = 0.32, 95% CI: 0.15 - 0.68) were mainly associated with luminal phenotype A (Figs. 1 and 2). The 'nucleolus' criterion also made it possible to distinguish luminal phenotype A from luminal phenotype B (OR = 2.99, 95% CI: 1.39 - 6.41) and showed marginal significance for differentiating luminal phenotype B from non-luminal phenotypes (OR = 3.73, 95% CI: 0.94 -14.82) (Table 4).

Table 2. Frequencies of the five cytological criteria in 169 FNABs, by molecular phenotype.

Variable	Category	Molecular phenotype			
		Luminal A	Luminal B	HER2 overexp.	Triple negative
Cellularity	Low	13(12.2%)	3 (7.7%)	0 (0.0%)	0 (0.0%)
	Moderate	29(27.1%)	14(35.9%)	1 (12.5%)	1 (6.7%)
	High	65 (60.7%)	22 (56.4%)	7 (87.5%)	14(93.3%)
Cell cohesion	Low	49 (45.8%)	24 (61.5%)	6 (75.0%)	10(66.7%)
	Moderate	48 (44.9%)	9(23.1%)	2 (25.0%)	4 (26.6%)
	High	10(9.3%)	6 (15.4%)	0 (0.0%)	1 (6.7%)

Necrosis	Present	64 (59.8%)	28 (71.8%)	8 (100.0%)	15(100.0%)
	Absent	43 (40.2%)	11 (28.2%)	0 (0.0%)	0 (0.0%)
Nucleolus	Inconspicuous	21 (19.6%)	6 (15.4%)	0 (0.0%)	0 (0.0%)
	Present	46 (43.0%)	8 (20.5%)	1 (12.5%)	2 (13.3%)
	Present and imminent	40 (37.4%)	25 (64.1%)	7 (87.5%)	13(86.7%)
Nuclear atypia	Lightweight	24 (22.4%)	4 (10.3%)	0 (0.0%)	0 (0.0%)
	Moderate	28 (26.2%)	9(23.1%)	1 (12.5%)	1 (6.7%)
	Intense	55 (51.4%)	26 (66.6%)	7 (87.5%)	14(93.3%)

Table 3. Frequency of markers in the TMA carried out on 169 breast cancer cases.

Molecular phenotype	ER		PR		HER2		Ki67*		E-cadherin	
	Negative	Positive	Negative	Positive	Negative	Positive	Low	Hlgti	Negative	Positive
Luminal A	0 (0.0%)	107 (63.3%)	24 (14.2%)	83 (49.1%)	107 (63.3%)	0 (0.0%)	107 (63.3%)	0 (0.0%)	58 (34.3%)	49 (29.0%)
Luminal B	0 (0.0%)	39 (23.1%)	17(10.1%)	22(13.0%)	26 (15.4%)	13(7.7%)	3(1.8%)	36 (21.3%)	14 (8.3%)	25 (14.8%)
HER2-overexpression	8 (4.7%)	0 (0.0%)	8 (4.7%)	0 (0.0%)	0 (0.0%)	8 (4.7%)	3(1.8%)	5 (3.0%)	0 (0.0%)	8 (47%)
Triple negative	15 (8.9%)	0 (0.0%)	15(8.9%)	0 (0.0%)	15(8.9%)	0 (0.0%)	6 (3.5%)	9 (5.3%)	0 (0.0%)	15(8.9%)
Total	23 (13.6%)	146 (86.4%)	64 (37.9%)	105 (62.1%)	146 (87.6%)	21 (12.4%)	119(70.4%)	50 (29.6%)	72 (42.6%)	97 (57.4%)

The 20 per cent *cut-off* was accepted by the *13th St Gallen Consensus Conference.*

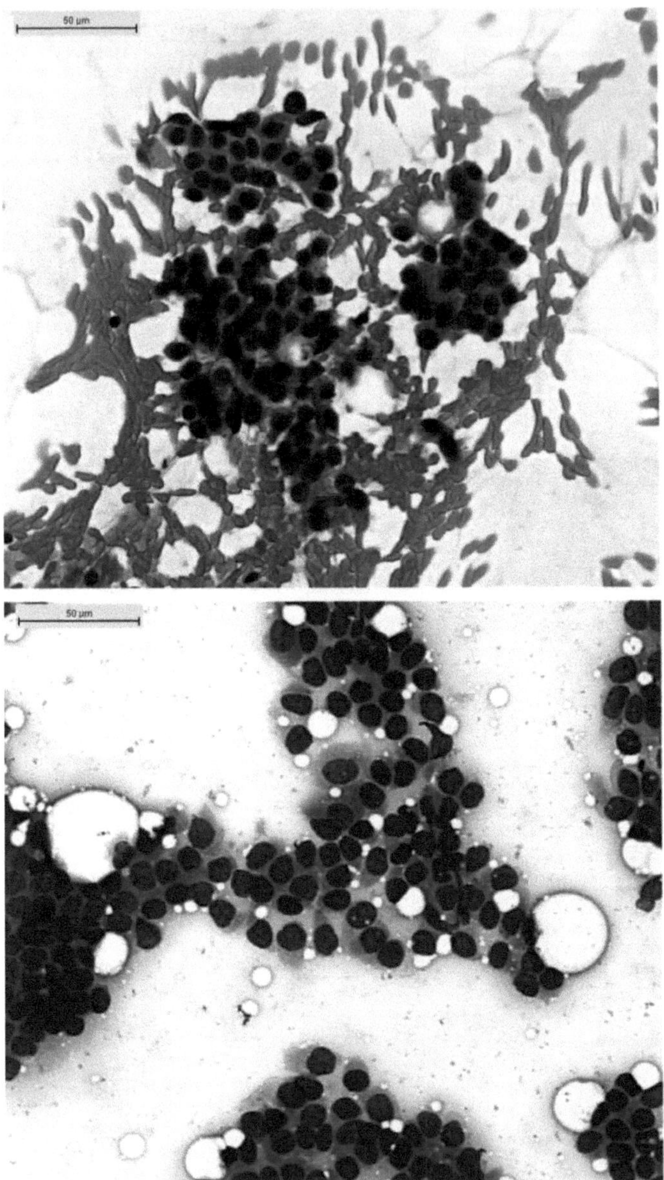

Figs. 1 and 2. Cell cohesion (HE; x400) and absence of necrosis (Giemsa; x400) were mainly associated with the Luminal A phenotype in FNACs.

Table 4. Association between the five cytological criteria and the different molecular phenotypes of breast cancer in 169 FNACs.

Cytological criteria	p-value	*OR* (95%CI)
Cellularity (low/moderate vs. high)		
Luminal vs Non-luminal	**0.010**	7.12(1.61 -31.52)
Luminal A x Non-luminal	**0.012**	6.78 (1.51 -30.45)
Luminal B x Non-luminal	**0.009**	8.11 (1.61 -39.49)
Luminal A x Luminal B	0.637	0.84 (0.40 - 1.76)
Luminal A x Other (including luminal B)	0.263	1.46 (0.75-2.84)
Cell cohesion (low vs. moderate/high)		
Luminal vs Non-luminal	0.087	0.44 (0.17-1.13)
Luminal A x Non-luminal	**0.043**	0.37 (0.14-0.97)
Luminal B x Non-luminal	0.524	0.70 (0.23-2.10)
Luminal A x Luminal B	0.095	0.53 (0.25-1.12)
Luminal A x Other (including luminal B)	**0.002**	0.46 (0.24 - 0.88)
Necrosis (present)		
Luminal vs Non-luminal	0.935	0.00 (0.00 - 999.99)
Luminal A x Non-luminal	0.934	0.00 (0.00 - 999.99)
Luminal B x Non-luminal	0.955	0.00 (0.00 - 999.99)
Luminal A x Luminal B	0.187	0.56 (0.26 - 1.30)
Luminal A x Other (including luminal B)	**0.003**	0.32 (0.15-0.68)
Nucleolus (inconspicuous/present vs. prominent)		
Luminal vs Non-luminal	**0.001**	8.31 (2.36-29.19)
Luminal A x Non-luminal	**0.000**	11.12 (3.12-39.94)
Luminal B x Non-luminal	0.061	3.73 (0.94-14.82)
Luminal A x Luminal B	**0.005**	2.99 (1.39-6.41)
Luminal A x Other (including luminal B)	**0.000**	4.43 (2.24 - 8.77)
Nuclear atypia (mild/moderate vs. intense)		
Luminal vs Non-luminal	**0.005**	8.42 (1.90-37.25)
Luminal A x Non-luminal	**0.003**	9.93 (2.22 - 44.44)
Luminal B x Non-luminal	**0.042**	5.25 (1.06-25.88)
Luminal A x Luminal B	0.103	1.89 (0.88-4.07)
Luminal A x Other (including luminal B)	**0.002**	2.96 (1.48-5.93)

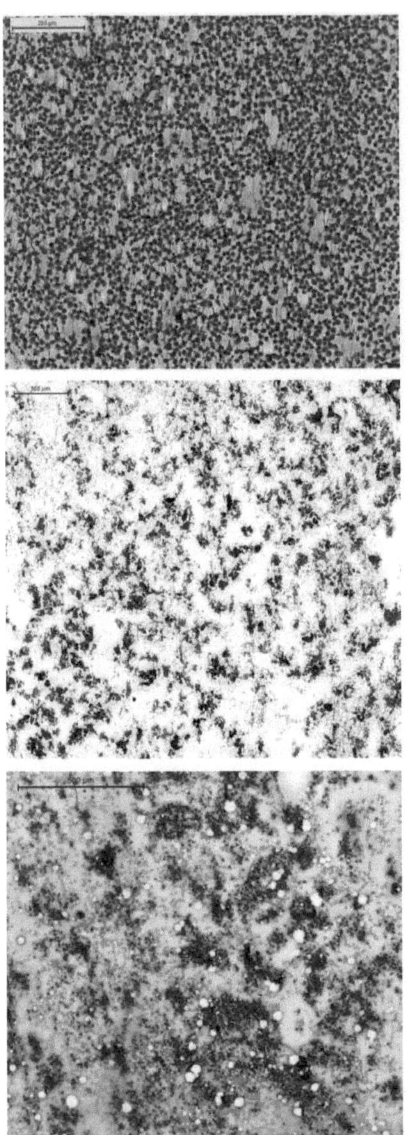

Figs. 3, 4 and 5. Cellularity assessment carried out at lower magnification (x100). The three stains used (HE, PAP and Giemsa) showed high cellularity. This criterion was mainly associated with the non-luminal phenotype of breast cancer.

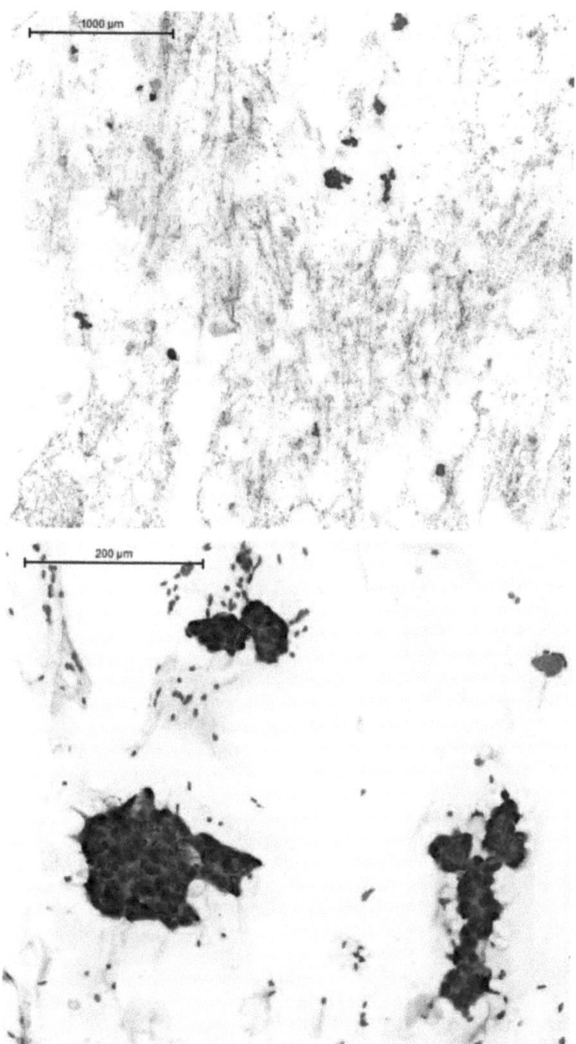

Figs. 6 and 7. Sample with low cellularity (HE, x25) also showing few cohesive clusters (HE, x200), cytological criteria that can be associated with the luminal phenotype of breast cancer.

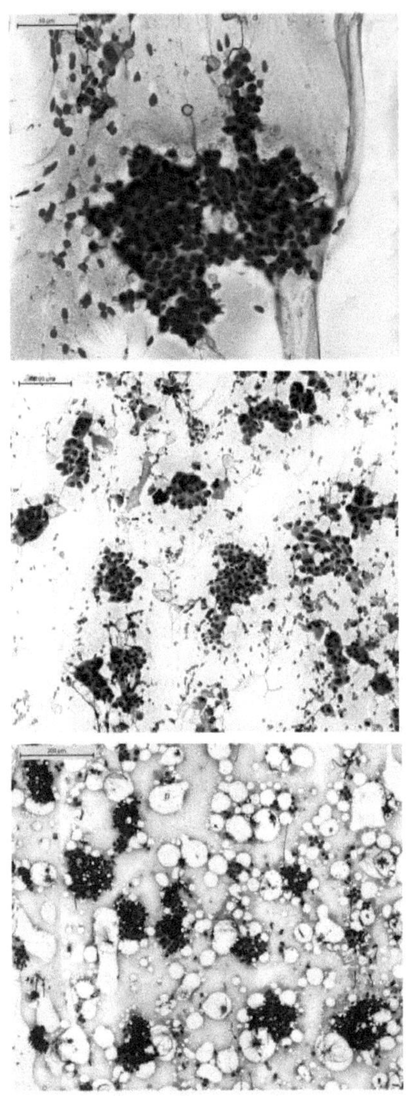

Figs. 8, 9 and 10: The evaluation of the 'cell cohesion' criterion can be satisfactorily carried out by the three stains used (Giemsa, PAP and HE, x200), showing groupings that are still cohesive. Reduced cell cohesion is a characteristic significantly associated with an increased risk of malignancy.

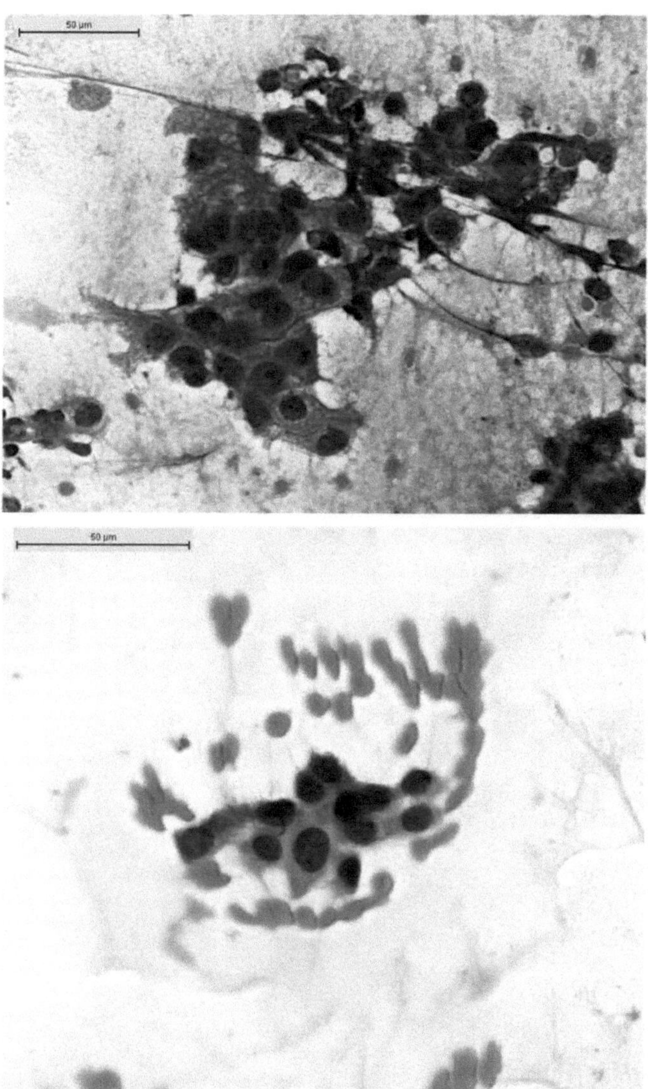

Figs. 11 and 12: The 'prominent nucleolus' criterion is more frequent for both the luminal B and non-luminal phenotypes (above) compared to luminal A, which in turn is routinely associated with inconspicuous nucleoli (below) (HE, x400).

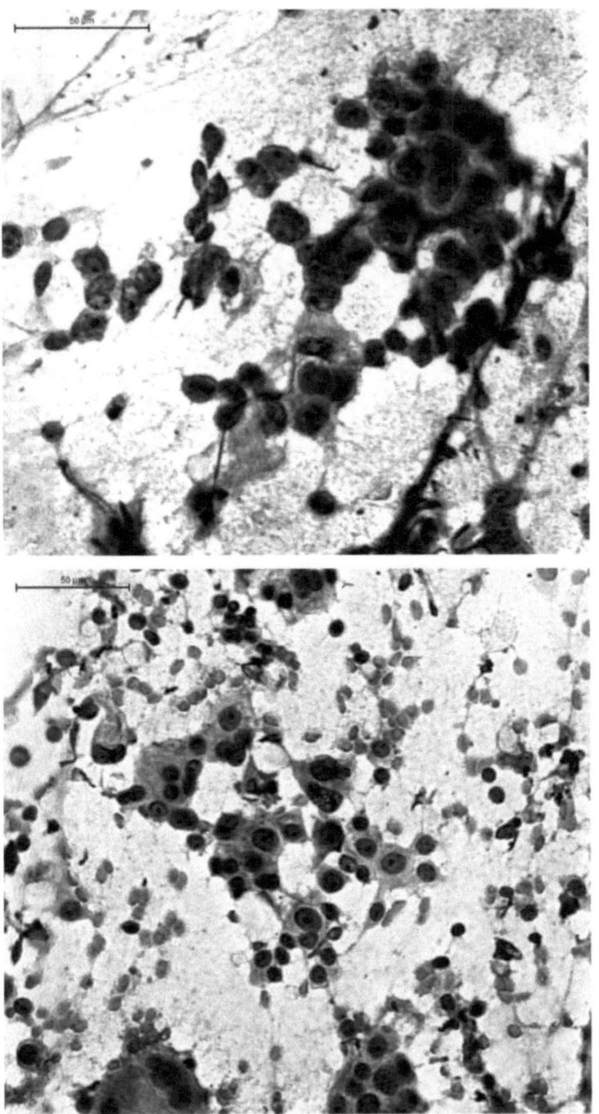

Figs. 13 and 14: Papanicolaou stain is preferred for identifying nuclear details, allowing better characterisation of the nucleolus and the degree of nuclear atypia (PAP, x400).

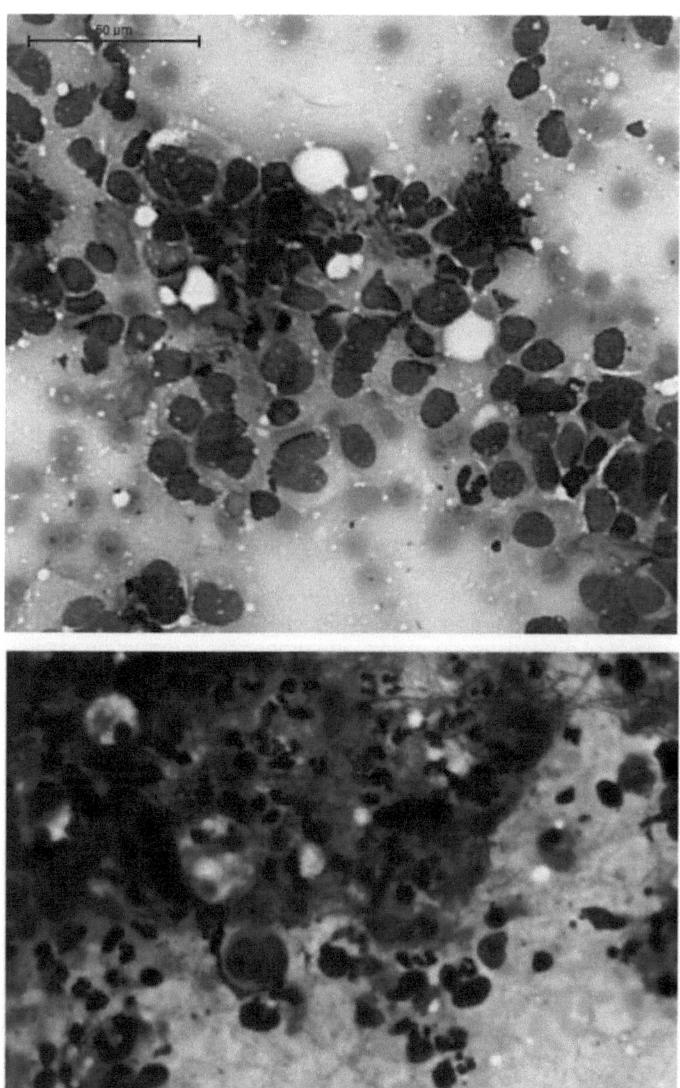

Figs. 15 and 16: Giemsa provides less nuclear detail than HE and PAP stains. Above, the presence of polymorphonuclear cells may be an indication of necrosis - a cytological criterion often associated with the basal phenotype of breast cancer, but unexpected for the luminal phenotype (Giemsa, x400).

CHAPTER 5

Discussion

In the era of personalised medicine, cytopathological specimens have gained in importance because they allow numerous molecular tests to be carried out, made possible above all by the adequate preservation and purity of the samples. These include DNA extraction techniques, next generation sequencing, proteomic studies, polymerase chain reaction and *in situ* hybridisation (Gailey et al., 2015; Wei et al., 2015; Knoepp et al., 2013). The paraffin embedding *(ce//block)* of the material obtained from the aspiration puncture makes it possible to perform immunocytochemistry and, therefore, the phenotypic characterisation of breast carcinoma. Thus, making a *cell block* is a routine practice whose intrinsic potential to gather a set of diagnostic, predictive and prognostic information in each case is closely related to the experience of the cytopathologist, avoiding additional diagnostic procedures (Collins et aL, 2015; Jain et aL, 2014).

Studies in the literature on the cytological criteria associated with the molecular phenotypes of breast carcinoma in FNAB are limited to the basal phenotype, whose most relevant criterion has been described as 'necrosis' (Dufloth et aL, 2009). To date, no study has set out to assess which cytological criteria could predict the luminal phenotype of breast cancer.

The investigation of five cytological criteria routinely applied by cytopathologists when analysing FNAB samples showed that the luminal phenotype tended to present less cellular smears than the non-luminal phenotypes, which was also well observed, at lower magnification, through the three stains used (Giemsa, PAP and HE) (Figs. 3, 4 and 5 and Figs. 6 and 7). Cell aggregates were also observed and, statistically, especially for the luminal phenotype A, there was greater cell cohesion compared to the other phenotypes (Figs. 8, 9 and 10).

Reduced cell cohesion is a characteristic significantly associated with an increased risk of malignancy. Wakasa and colleagues (Wakasa et aL, 2014) described a subclassification for breast cytology with loss of cell cohesion, and for invasive lobular carcinoma, medullary carcinoma, neuroendocrine carcinoma and solid papillary carcinoma this criterion was present in the majority of cases. However, the 'cell cohesion' criterion has not yet been studied in breast carcinoma with a luminal phenotype.

With regard to the 'absence of necrosis' criterion, there was statistical significance in distinguishing luminal phenotype A from the others. According to the literature, this phenotype generally has a lower nuclear grade, so the presence of extensive necrosis is not expected (Maisonneuve et aL, 2014; Badve et aL, 2011). Incidentally, the luminal B phenotype is related to the presence of a higher nuclear grade (Creighton et aL, 2012; Cheang et aL, 2009), which may require further evaluation of nuclear details.

The presence of prominent nucleoli was statistically remarkable for both the luminal B and non-luminal phenotypes compared to luminal A (Figs. 11 and 12). However, we are aware of the limitations of establishing subjective size parameters for assessing nucleoli. In this regard, cytomorphometry in computerised images of breast FNAC samples has been described as an auxiliary tool, with highly objective parameters (Yadav et aL, 2015). It is hoped that this technique will also be applied to the identification of specific breast cancer phenotypes.

There is discussion in the literature about the preferred staining methods for breast cytology (Anand et al., 2004; Cibas et al., 2009). Giemsa seems to be associated with fewer technical problems, better accuracy, sensitivity and specificity compared to HE and PAP, which in turn is especially useful for assessing nuclear characteristics as well as cytoplasmic differentiation (Cibas et al., 2009) (Figs. 13 and 14) (Figs. 15 and 16).

The comparison of staining methods has already been researched in the assessment of breast cancer metastases in lymph nodes using cytological *imprinting* in intraoperative examination (Anand et aL, 2004), but remains an encouraging subject for future cytomorphological studies applied to breast cancer phenotyping.

The differentiation of the luminal phenotype of breast cancer, especially luminal A, is of clinical interest, since this phenotype has a better prognosis and is associated with lower mortality and mestastasis rates (Falck et al., 2013), but may also be associated with lobular carcinoma, according to recent studies (Ciriello et al., 2015).

CHAPTER 6

Conclusion

To date, no study has been identified that investigates the individual cytological criteria that could identify the luminal phenotype of breast carcinoma.

1. In terms of frequency, the cytological smears obtained by FNAB of luminal breast carcinomas showed low and moderate cellularity (40.4%), inconspicuous nucleoli or those present but not prominent (55.5%) and mild to moderate nuclear atypia (44.5%).

2. With regard to the association of the cytological criteria for the luminal phenotype of breast carcinoma, the cytological smears showed low and moderate cellularity (OR = 7.12, 95%CI: 1.61 - 31.52), inconspicuous nucleoli or nucleoli present but not prominent (OR = 8.31, 95%CI: 2.36 - 29.19) and mild to moderate nuclear atypia (OR = 8.42, 95%CI: 1.90 - 37.25). The luminal A phenotype was associated with less loss of cell cohesion (OR = 0.46, 95%CI: 0.24 - 0.88), showing clusters with moderate to intense cell cohesion, and absence of necrosis (OR = 0.32, 95%CI: 0.15 - 0.68), and the cytological criterion 'nucleolus' also made it possible to distinguish luminal A and luminal B phenotypes (OR = 2.99, 95%CI: 1.39 - 6.41).

Further research is needed with larger samples and the application of new molecular markers possibly related to the luminal phenotype, in order to find out which cytological, predictive and prognostic criteria are related to this phenotype in cytological smears obtained by FNAB. The difficulties are considerable, given the genetic and molecular heterogeneity associated with this phenotype.

The application of predictive cytological criteria in the daily routine of FNAB could lead to the development of possible diagnostic models with greater precision and accuracy, with the aim of establishing an early diagnosis and prompt therapeutic management of patients with breast carcinoma.

CHAPTER 7

Bibliographical references

Aleksandarany MA et al. Prognostic value of proliferation assay in the luminal, HER2-positive, and triple-negative biologic classes of breast cancer. Breast Cancer Research. 2012; 14(1)R3.

American Cancer Society. Cancer Facts & Figures 2017. American Cancer Society; 2017.

Anand M, Kumar R, Jain P, Asthana S, Deo SV, Shukla NK, Karak A: Comparison of three different staining techniques for intraoperative assessment of nodal metastasis in breast cancer. Diagn CytopatholL 2004; 31:423-426.

Andrade VP, Cunha IW, Silva EM, Ayala F, Sato Y, Ferreira SS, Nascimento CF, Soares FA. Tissue microarrays: high throughput and low cost available for pathologists. J Bras Patol Med Lab. 2007; 43(1):55-60.

Arisio R, Cuccorese C, Accinelli G, Mano MP, Bordon R, Fessia L. Role of fine- needle aspiration biopsy in breast lesions: analysis of a series of 4,110 cases. Diagn CytopatholL 1998; 18(6):462-7.

Badve S, Dabbs DJ, et al. Basal-like and triple-negative breast cancers: a critical review with an emphasis on the implications for pathologists and oncologists. Modern Pathology. 2011; 24:157-167.

Banerjee S, Reis-Filho JS, et al. Basal-like breast carcinomas: clinical outcome and response to chemotherapy. J Clin PatholL 2006; 59:729-735.

Bartsch R. et al. Present and future breast cancer management-bench to bedside and back: a positioning paper of academia, regulatory authorities and pharmaceutical industry. Ann OncolL 2013; 1-8 201.

Baselga J, Campone M, Piccart M et al. Everolimus in postmenopausal hormone receptor-positive advanced breast cancer. N Engl J Med. 2012; 366: 520-529.

Bibbo M, Wilbur D. Comprehensive Cytopathology, Breast. 3(rd) edition. Philadelphia,

Saunders Elsevier. 2008; 715.

Billgren AM, Tani E, Liedberg A, Skoog L, Rutqvist LE. Prognostic significance of tumour cell proliferation analysed in fine needle aspirates from primary breast cancer. Breast Cancer Res Treat. 2002; 71 (2): 161-170.

Blows FM, Driver KE, Schmidt MK, Broeks A, Van Leeuwen FE, Wesseling J, Cheang MC, Gelmon K, Nielsen TO, Blomqvist C, et al. Subtyping of breast cancer by immunohistochemistry to investigate a relationship between subtype and short and long term survival: a collaborative analysis of data for 10,159 cases from 12 studies. PLoS Med. 2010; 7(5):e1000279.

Bose S. Triple-negative breast carcinoma: morphologic and molecular subtypes. Adv Anat PatholL 2015; 22(5):306-313.

Callagy G, Cattaneo E, Daigo Y, Happerfield L, Bobrow LG, Pharoah PD, Caídas C. Molecular classification of breast carcinomas using tissue microarrays. Diagn Mol PatholL 2003; 12(1):27-34.

Cancer Genome Atlas Network. Comprehensive molecular portraits of human breast tumours. Nature. 2012; 4;490(7418):61-70.

Chaiwun B, Thorner P. Fine needle aspiration for evaluation of breast masses. Curr Opin Obstet and GynecoL 2007; 19(1):48-55.

Cheang MC, Chia SK, Voduc D, Gao D, Leung S, Snider J, Watson M, Davies S, Bernard PS, Parker JS, et al. Ki67 index, HER2 status, and prognosis of patients with luminal B breast cancer. J Natl Cancer Inst. 2009; 101(10)736-50.

Cibas ES, Ducatman BS. Cytology: Principies and Clinical Correlates, ed 3. Philadelphia, Saunders Elsevier. 2009; pp 221-227.

Ciriello G, et al. Comprehensive molecular portraits of invasive lobular breast cancer. Cell. 2015; 163:506-19.

Coates AS, Winer EP, et al. Tailoring therapies - improving the management of early breast cancer: St Gallen International Expert Consensus on the Primary Therapy of Early Breast Cancer. Ann OncoL 2015; 26:1533-46.

Collins BT, Garcia TC, Hudson JB. Effective clinicai practices for improved FNA biopsy cell block outcomes. Cancer Cytopathology 2015; 123(9):540-7.

Creighton CJ. The molecular profile of luminal B breast cancer. Biologics: Targets and Therapy. 2012; 6: 289-97.

DeMay M. Practical principies of cytopathology. Revised Edition. American Society for Clinical Pathology. 2007; 257-80.

Di Lorito A, Schmitt FC. (Cyto)pathology and sequencing: Next (or last) generation? Diagn CytopathoL 2011; 40(5)459-61.

Dufloth RM, Alves JM, Martins D, et aL Cytological criteria to predict basal phenotype of breast carcinomas. Diagn CytopathoL 2009; 37:809-14.

Dufloth RM, Xavier-Júnior JCC, Neto FAM, Santos KJ, Schmitt F. Fine needle aspiration cytology of lobular breast carcinoma and its variants. Acta CytoL 2015; 59:37-42.

Eisenberg AJ, Hajdu SI, Winhelmus J, Melamed MR, Kinne D. Preoperative aspiration cytology of breast tumours. Acta CytoL 1986; 30(2): 135-46.

Esposito A, et aL Highlights from the 14th St Gallen International Breast Cancer Conference 2015 in Vienna: Dealing with classification, prognostication, and prediction refinement to personalise the treatment of patients with early breast cancer. Ecancer. 2015; 9:518.

Fadare O, Tavassoli FA. The phenotypic spectrum of basal-like breast cancers: a critical appraisaL Adv Anat PathoL 2007; 14(5):358-373.

Falck AK, et aL St Gallen molecular subtypes in primary breast cancer and matched lymph node metastases - aspects on distribution and prognosis for patients with luminal A tumours: results from a prospective randomized trial. BMC Cancer. 2013; 13:558.

Gailey MP, Stence AA et aL Multiplatform comparison of molecular oncology tests performed on cytology specimens and formalin-fixed, paraffin-embedded tissue. Cancer Cytopathology 2015; 123(1):30-9.

Gerhard R, Carvalho A, Carneiro V, Bento RS, Uemura G, Gomes M, Albergaria A, Schmitt F. Clinicopathological significance of ERCC1 expression in breast cancer. Pathol Res Pract. 2013; 206(6):331-6.

Geyer FC et al. Molecular classification of estrogen receptor-positive/luminal breast cancers. Adv Anat Pathol. 2012; 19(1):39-53.

Goldhirsch A, Winer EP, Coates AS, Gelber RD, Piccart-Gebhart M, Thurlimann B, et al. Personalising the treatment of women with early breast cancer: highlights of the St Gallen International Expert Consensus on the Primary Therapy of Early Breast Cancer 2013. Ann OncoL 2013;24:2206-23.

Goldhirsch A, Wood WC, Coates AS, Gelber RD, Thurlimann B, Senn HJ, et al. Strategies for subtypes: dealing with the diversity of breast cancer: highlights of the St. Gallen International Expert Consensus on the Primary Therapy of Early Breast Cancer 2011. Ann OncoL 2011 ;22:1736^17.

Hammond MEH, et aL American Society of Clinical Oncology/College of American Pathologists recommendations for immunohistochemical testing of estrogen and progesterone receptors in breast cancer. J Clin OncoL 2010; 28(16):2784-95.

Hwang S, loffe O, Lee I, Waisman J, Cangiarella J, Simsir A. Cytologic diagnosis of invasive lobular carcinoma: factors associated with negative and equivocal diagnoses. Diagn CytopathoL 2004; 31:87-93.

National Cancer Institute (Brazil). Estimativa 2016: incidência de câncer no Brasil /Instituto Nacional de Câncer José Alencar Gomes da Silva, Coordenação Geral de Ações Estratégicas, Coordenação de Prevenção e Vigilância. - Rio de Janeiro: INCA; 2015.

National Cancer Institute [Internet]. Brazil: Portal do Instituto Nacional de Câncer [updated in 2017; cited in 2015 Nov 10 (access 05/06/17)]. Available from: http://www2.inca.gov.br/wps/wcm/connect/tiposdecancer/site/home/mama/cancer_m ama

Jain D, Mathur SR, Iyer VK. Cell blocks in cytopathology: a review of preparative methods, utility in diagnosis and role in ancillary studies. Cytopathology. 2014;

25:356-71.

Jayaram G, Elsayed EM. Cytologic evaluation of prognostic markers in breast carcinoma. Acta CytoL 2005; 49(6):605-10.

Kamphausen BH, Toellner T, Ruschenburg I. The value of ultrasound-guided fine-needle aspiration cytology of the breast: 354 cases with cytohistological correlation. Anticancer Res. 2003; 23(3C):3009-13.

Karimzadeh M, Sauer T. Diagnostic accuracy of fine-needle aspiration cytology in histological grade 1 breast carcinomas: are we good enough? Cytopathology 2008; 19(5):279-86.

Knoepp SM, Roh MH. Ancillary techniques on direct-smear aspirate slides: a significant evolution for cytopathology techniques. Cancer Cytopathology 2013; 121 (3): 120-8.

Kocjan G et aL Fine needle aspiration cytology: a survey of current European practice. CytopatholL 2006; 17(5):219-26.

Kocjan G et aL The role of breast FNAC in diagnosis and clinical management: a survey of current practice. Cytopathology. 2008; 19(5):271-8.

Kohler BA, Recinda L et aL Annual report to the nation on the status of cancer, 1975- 2011, featuring incidence of breast cancer subtypes by race/ethnicity, poverty, and State. JNCI J Natl Cancer Inst. 2015; 107(6)djv048.

Koss LG. Koss's diagnostic cytology. 5 th ed. Philadelphia, PA: Lippincott Williams & Wilkins; 2006; 1004-1120.

Koss LG. The palpable breast nodule: a cost-effectiveness analysis of alternate diagnostic approaches. The role of the needle aspiration biopsy. Cancer. 1993; 72 (5): 1499-502.

Lakhani SR, Ellis IO, Schnitt SJ, Tan PH, Van De Vijver MJ. World Health Organization Classification of Tumours of the Breast. Lyon, France: IARC Press; 4th edition. 2012; 34^2.

Layfield LJ, Chrischilles EA, Cohen MB, Bottles K. The palpable breast nodule: A cost-effectiveness analysis of alternate diagnostic approaches. Cancer. 1993; 72(5): 1642-51.

Lõfgren L, Skoog L, Von Schoultz E, Tani E, Isaksson E, Fernstad R, Carlstrõm K, Von Schoultz B. Hormone receptor status in breast cancer - a comparison between surgical specimens and fine needle aspiration biopsies. Cytopathology. 2003; 14(3): 136-142.

Lowery AJ, Kell MR, Glynn RW et al. Locoregional recurrence after breast cancer surgery: a systematic review by receptor phenotype. Breast Cancer Res Treat. 2012; 133:831-841.

Maisonneuve P, Disalvatore D, et al. Proposed new clinicopathological surrogate definitions of luminal A and luminal B (HER2-negative) intrinsic breast cancer subtypes. Breast Cancer Research. 2014; 16:R65.

Marinsek ZP, Nolde N, Kardum-Skelin I, Nizzoli R, Onal B, Rezanko T, Tani E, Ostovic KT,

Vielh P, Schmitt F, Kocjan G. Multinational study of oestrogen and progesterone receptor immunocytochemistry on breast carcinoma fine needle aspirates. CytopathoL 2013; 24(1):7-20.

Marsan C, Adotti F et al. Cytopathologie mammaire par ponction. Le pathologiste. Elsevier. 2001.

Martin H, Ellis E. Biopsy by needle puncture and aspiration. Ann Surg. 1930; 92(2): 169-81.

Naderi A, Teschendorff AE, Barbosa-Morais NL, Pinder SE, Green AR, Powe DG, Robertson JF, Aparicio S, Ellis IO, Brenton JD, Caídas C: A gene- expression signature to predict survival in breast cancer across independent data sets. Oncogene 2007; 26:1507-16.

Neto FAM. Analysis of the clinical relevance of the histological classification of lobular breast carcinomas and its relationship with the molecular classification [master's thesis]. Botucatu. Botucatu School of Medicine. Universidade Estadual Paulista; 2014.

Perou CM, Sorlie T, Eisen MB, Van de Rijn M, Jeffrey SS, Rees CA, et aL Molecular portraits of human breast tumours. Nature. 2000. 17; 406(6797):747-52.

Pessoa CPKC. Correlation of ultrasound characteristics with the immunohistochemical profile of malignant breast tumours [PhD thesis]. Botucatu. Botucatu School of Medicine. Universidade Estadual Paulista; 2014.

Rakha E, et aL Basal-like breast cancer: a critical review. J Clin OncoL 2008; 26(5)15:2568-81.

Schmitt FC, Soares R, Leitão D. Detection of numerical chromosome 17 abnormalities in fine-needle aspirates of breast cancer using a novel in situ hybridisation signal amplification method. Diagn Cytopath. 1997; 19(2):141-46.

Schmitt FC et aL Molecular biology and cytopathology. Principies and applications. Annales de pathologie. 2012; 32(1)57-63.

Schmitt FC, Longatto-Filho A, Valent A, Vielh P. Molecular techniques in cytopathology practice. J Clin Pathol 2008;61:258-267.

Shabb NS, Boulos FI, Abdul-Karim FW. Indeterminate and erroneous fine-needle aspirates of breast with focus on the 'true grey zone': a review. Acta Cytol 2013; 57:316-331.

Sikora MJ, Cooper KL, Bahreini A, Luthra S, Wang G, Chandran UR, Davidson NE, Dabbs DJ, Welm AL, Oesterreich S. Invasive lobular carcinoma cell lines are characterised by unique estrogen-mediated gene expression patterns and altered tamoxifen response. Cancer Res. 2014; 74:1463-1474.

Sorlie T, Perou CM, Tibshirani R, Aas T, Geisler S, Johnsen H, et aL Gene expression patterns of breast carcinomas distinguish tumour subclasses with clinical implications. Proc Natl Acad Sei USA. 2001; 98(19): 10869-74.

Sorlie T, Perou CM, Tibshirani R, Parker J, Hastie T, Marron JS, Nobel A, et aL Repeated observation of breast tumour subtypes in independent gene expression data sets. Proc Natl Acad Sei USA. 2003; 00(14):8418-23.

Sotiriou C, Wirapati P, Loi S, Harris A, Fox S, Smedes J, et aL Gene expression profiling in breast cancer: understanding the molecular basis of histologic grade to improve prognosis. J Natl Cancer Inst. 2006; 15;98(4):262-72.

Stanley MW, Sidawy MK, Sanchez MA, Stahl RE, Goldfisher M. Current issues in breast cytopathology. Am J Cin Pathol. 2000; 113(5)49-75.

Tabchy A, Valero V, Vidaurre T, Lluch A, Gomez H, Martin M, et al. Evaluation of a 30-gene paclitaxel, fluorouracil, doxorubicin, and cyclophosphamide chemotherapy response predictor in a multicentre randomized trial in breast cancer. Clin Cancer Res 2010;16:5351-61.

Tan SM, Behranwala KA, Trott PA, et al. A retrospective study comparing the individual modalities of triple assessment in the pre-operative diagnosis of invasive lobular breast carcinoma. Eur J Surg OncoL 2002; 28:203-208.

Van't Veer LJ, Dai H, Van de Vijver MJ, He YD, Hart AA, Mao M, et aL Gene expression profiling predicts clinicai outcome of breast cancer. Nature. 2002; 415(6871):530-6.

Wakasa T, Nakamura M, et aL Loss of cellular cohesion in cytology composes a special subgroup of breast tumours - analyses of 37 cases. Acta CytoL 2014; 58(1):89-95.

Wei S et aL Using "residual" FNA rinse and body fluid specimens for next-generation sequencing: An institutional experience. Cancer Cytopathology 2015; doi:10.1002/cncy.21666.

Wolff A, et aL Recommendations for Human Epidermal Growth Factor Receptor 2 testing in breast cancer. ASCO/CAP Clinical Practice Guideline Update. Arch Pathol Med Lab. 2013.

Yadav H, Gill M, Srivastava D, Gupta V, Sen R: Significance of morphometric parameters in the categorisation of breast lesions on cytology. Turk Patoloji Derg. 2015; 31:188-193.

Zagorianakou P, Fiaccavento S, Zagorianakou N, Makrydimas G, Stefanou D, Agnantis NJ. FNAC: its role, limitations and perspective in the preoperative diagnosis

of breast cancer. Eur J Gynaecol OncoL 2005; 26(2):143-9.

Zhang L, Li J et aL Identifying ultrasound and clinical features of breast cancer molecular subtypes by ensemble decision. Nature. Scientific Reports. 2015; 5:11085.

ANNEXES

Data collection form

DATA COLLECTION FORM

1. **Case number:**
2. **Paraffin block number:**
3. **Aspiration puncture number:**
4. **Breast carcinoma phenotypes:**
    - **4.1.** Luminal A
    - **4.2.** Luminal B
    - **4.3.** HER2 overexpression
    - **4.4.** Triple negative

4.5. Mobile phones:
- 1 = Discrete
- 2= Moderate
- 3= Accentuated

4.6. Cell cohesion:
- 1= Little
- 2= Moderate
- 3= Accentuated

4.7. Necrosis:
- 1 = Present
- 2= Absent

4.8. Nucleolus:
- 1= Inconspicuous
- 2= Present
- 3= Present and prominent

4.9. Nuclear atypia:
- 1 = Absent
- 2= Discrete
- 3= Moderate

4= Intense

Tissue microarray (TMA) spreadsheet

Observer: ( ) 1 ( ) 2
TMA PLAN ____

Case number	E-cadherin	Ki67	RE	PR	HER2

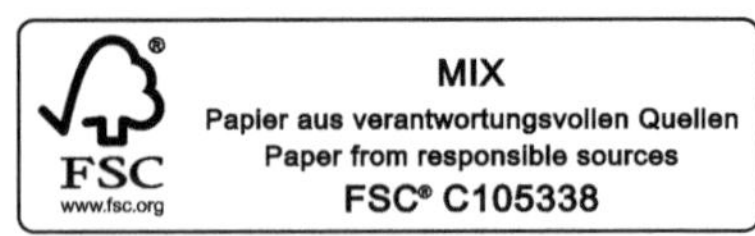

Printed by Books on Demand GmbH, Norderstedt / Germany